I0439421

INTRODUCTION

The object of this book is to provide clear and complete information on the subject of traditional wet shaving and shaving with a straight razor. I have found there are many men who, for various reasons, are not happy with their current shaving method and are interested in learning how to shave with a straight razor. I understand that many people in this day and age of austerity are finding themselves under financial pressure and are looking for ways to save money.

I also understand that the art of shaving and grooming in general is a subject, which, for reasons, is being neglected as knowledge to be taught to teenage boys by fathers' and/or the educational system in general. Experience has taught me that with proper knowledge shaving with a straight razor can yield better results, in terms of cost, comfort, environmental impact, and shaving results then almost any other method of shaving. These days many men see going to a barber for a straight razor shave as a luxury. However, I believe with basic information found in this book a man can indulge in this luxury in the privacy of his own home, using his own razor, cup, soap, towels, and brush, which he can keep scrupulously clean and sterile, thereby avoiding the risk of infection and blood born diseases and unlike a barber shop you don't have to wait to be 'next'.

The art of shaving with a straight razor with the basic

tools and some time can be easily acquired as long as one has the will.

This book has been designed to give the beginner all the basic information they need to learn this basic skill, which will last them a lifetime.

I believe if instructions in this book are carefully read and applied, then with a little time and practice any beginner can master this skill and will be able to shave himself better.

Contents

What You Need To Get Started

You will need top-quality tools from the beginning. Many beginners have given up on this pursuit because no matter how hard they tried or how much they practiced they could never get satisfactory results, never knowing that while their technique was OK, the poor result was due to the poor tools they were using.

No matter how skillfully one can handle shaving tools, inferior tools will always yield poor results.

Many bad shaves have resulted from poor razors, hones, strops, and soaps as from lack of knowledge of how to use them.

Simply put, to get a good shave, good tools and the skill in using them must go hand in hand.
A good but very basic straight razor shaving kit should consist of:

- A good quality straight razor
- A top-quality strop
- A mirror
- A cup or shaving mug
- A cake of quality shaving soap
- And a bottle of quality aftershave lotion

These are the basic necessities however, even these may be added to as in time you may need:

- A good quality hone
- Talcum power
- And a septic pencil or other form of antiseptic

While the above three items are not absolutely necessary they will add much to the comfort, convenience, and luxury of shaving with a straight razor.

The Razor

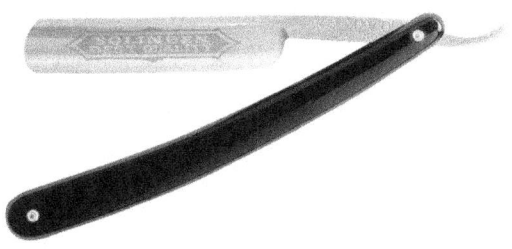

An excellent razor

Of course, the razor itself is the most important part of your straight razor shaving kit, and your success or failure depends largely on the type and quality of the razor you select.

Don't purchase a razor just because it's cheap, for shaving, a poor quality razor is expensive at any price. You want a good quality razor NOT a cheap razor.

A good quality razor will comfortably shave you for years and be a joy to use.

A poor quality razor will not shave properly (if at all) no matter how well you hone or strop it, and it will irritate the skin and be a source of continual trouble.

One of the main things to consider when selecting a razor is the type and quality of the steel used in the blade. Today there are many cheap razors being sold with the blade made of stainless steel, this in itself is a good sign you should leave this razor alone, the best straight razor blades are made of hardened steel, not stainless steel. What is meant by "quality" is the temper of steel or how solid the steel is, and if it is capable of receiving even after many year a fine edge. This is the first thing you should consider. But how do you judge the temper of a razor without trying it out? The human eye is not sufficient; it cannot see any of the major defects in the blade. The irregularities of a razor's edge, which are caused by poor workmanship or improper tempering, are usually so slight that they remain indistinguishable until the razor is used. They will, however, add extra friction to the skin whilst shaving, especially if the skin is thin and tender.

The easiest way to check the temper of a blade is to catch the point of the blade under your thumbnail and then let your nail slip off quickly. If the blade gives a good, clear ringing sound then you may rest assured that the blade is well tempered, but if it does not give a good, clear ring this indicates that the blade has been unevenly tempered.

It should be noted that a razor's blade is only as good as the quality of the blade's edge. If a razor's blade is too brittle as a result of being overheated whist being hardened or not cooled down enough whilst being tempered it will NEVER take a proper cutting edge regardless of how well it is honed or stropped.

Concave Blades

Most new straight razors today are made with hollow-ground blades. The main advantage of this design is that the thinnest blade edge is always the sharpest and, therefore, a blade's edge should be as thin as the metal itself will allow.

The other advantage is that a hollow ground blade is easier to sharpen.

Many blades are available as half, three quarters, or full concave. The full concave blade offers the thinnest edge, now you would think that full concave blade will offer the best shave. However, from my own observations this is not so. Because on a deeply ground razor the blade is extremely thin, the edge itself is almost paper thin. Unless such a blade is held very flat to the face such a blade may have a tenancy to flex and spring, may be difficult to shave with, and frequent nicks and cuts may result.

Point of Straight Razor Blade

The furthest point of a straight razor should be slightly rounded (unlike a Sweeney Todd razor) as shown in the following image.

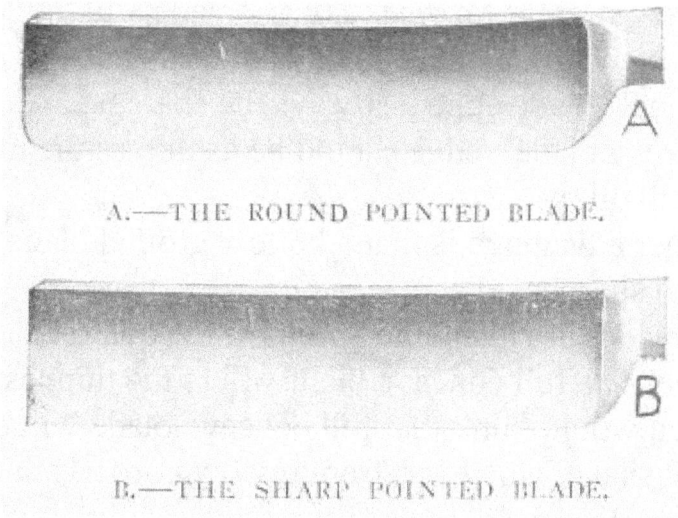

A.—THE ROUND POINTED BLADE.

B.—THE SHARP POINTED BLADE.

While this may not sound like a big deal but pointed blades do tend to cause more nicks. To round the edge of a hone, use the edge of the hone. NEVER use the main surface of the hone, as you may dig a scratch into the hone and ruin it, also make sure you use plenty of water so as to insure the blade doesn't over heat, as this may ruin the blade's temper.

Blade Width

Hollow-Ground razor blades are available in many widths; however, the four main widths are 3/8, 4/8, 5/8, and 7/8.

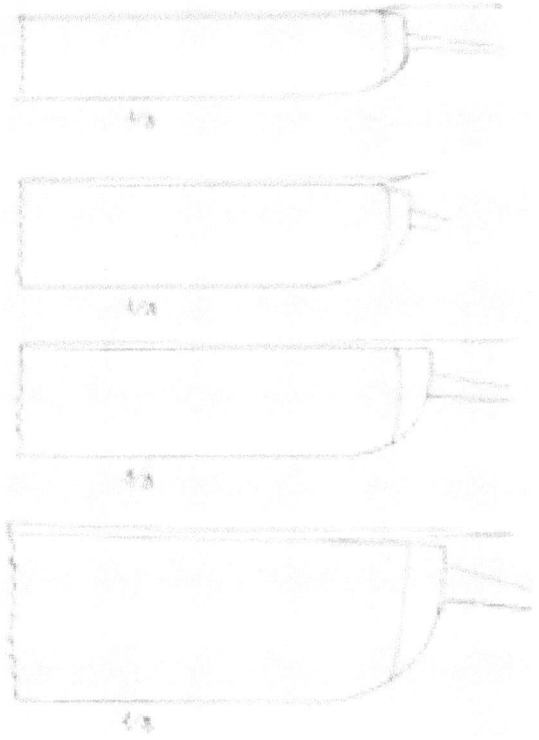

The above image shows the four main blade widths.

As a general rule a beginner should not start shaving with too wide a blade. As too wide a blade may be more awkward to handle and may flex and spring, which may lead to cuts or nicks. Ideally, a beginner should begin with 4/8 to 5/8 blade, as these blades are wide enough to follow the contours of the face, offer a very good shave, and is easier to handle.

Caring For Your Razor

 A quality straight razor is not cheap, which is why you should take care of your razor. A properly cared for razor should last the owner a lifetime. However the life will always depend entirely on the care it receives. Never store a razor until it has been properly dried. To dry, wipe the razor blade with a chamois or paper towel. Even this will not completely remove the moisture so it is recommended to let the razor air dry until all the moisture, which wasn't removed by the chamois, has evaporated. Make use there is no water between the scales. It is also good practice to apply a little oil to the blade to further prevent rusting; razor oil is ideal, however, any non-toxic oil such as vegetable oil will do. After these precautions have been taken you can safely put the razor back in its box and expect too find it in good condition when you next need to use it.

 Rusting must be prevented. Especially as the edges seem more prone to rusting than any other part of the blade. A tiny spot of rust on this delicate area will cause the metal to soften and crumble, and will soon negate the usefulness of the razor, when this happens the only remedy is to grind the blade back past the spot. In this case there is always the possibility of not getting a proper edge.

When wiping hair and lather off the blade don't use course paper.
A soft towel or paper towel is a much better option. Many men draw the blade straight across course paper, turn the edge, and wonder why the blade doesn't feel as sharp as it once did. Draw the blade over the towel obliquely, in the same direction as if you were stropping it.

Cartridge and Disposable Razors

For many years now most men have been using cartridge or disposable razors. The sales and marketing strategy pitch for these razors has been pretty consistent for a while now. Simply create a cartridge razor with one or two extra gimmicks that the previous models didn't have, e.g., a vibrating handle, a few extra blades, and different styling, sell the razor with say four extra cartridges to entice men to buy them and then hit them for expensive replacement cartridges when they'll soon need them. While these cartridge razors have a few advantages such as you are less likely to cut your self with them and, therefore, can shave quicker with them and because they are disposable they require no maintenance. The disadvantages vastly outweighs the advantages for instance most multiple blades are spaced very close together making it difficult to clean hair from between them and causing tugging and pulling at longer stubble (don't ever try to shave a beard with one).

  Many companies advertise a lubricating strip, which is supposed to help the razor "glide" over the skin, that strip usually wears out after the first two shaves making it a gimmick more then anything else.

The straight razor provides many advantages over the disposable razor including:

Closer, more comfortable shaves.

Unlike modern disposable razors and electric razors, the straight razor's blade actually touches the surface of the skin resulting in closer shaves and if done properly a straight razor shave can be the most comfortable shave available resulting in less skin irritation and less aftershave bumps, which is especially important for people shaving sensitive skin.

No blade blockage.

Do you have a beard or have you forgotten to shave for a few days? Well with a straight razor the hair goes over the face of the blade, which means you are not forever trying to unblock the razor or going over the facial hair with clippers first.

Reduced shaving cost.

Sure, the initial cost of buying everything you need to start shaving with a straight razor costs more than a good disposable razor, but after these initial investments you are set for life, aside from shaving foam you will not need to spend anything more to shave again. A straight razor is something that if kept in good condition can be passed on from father to son.

It's environmentally friendly.

Think of all the materials and energy that is wasted to produce disposable razor cartridges and think of the landfill needed to dispose of them. All this waste is eliminated as a quality straight razor, if properly maintained, will last a lifetime and will not need to be replaced.

Satisfaction.

There is nothing most men find more satisfying then mastering a life skill that most modern men haven't.

Great investment potential.

Easy to store and keep safe some vintage, rare, or one off razors, if kept in good condition, hold their value well and actually appreciate in value as the years progress. To see how well a quality vintage straight razor holds its value one only has to check on E bay. How much do you think an old Gillette Fusion razor will be worth in fifty years?

The Hone

If you had to view the edge of a straight razor under a microscope it would look very different then what you would see with your naked eye. To the naked eye the edge of a straight razor appears as a continuous shiny line. However, this is not actually the case, under a microscope the edge is actually composed of thousands of microscopic teeth similar to a hack saw blade.

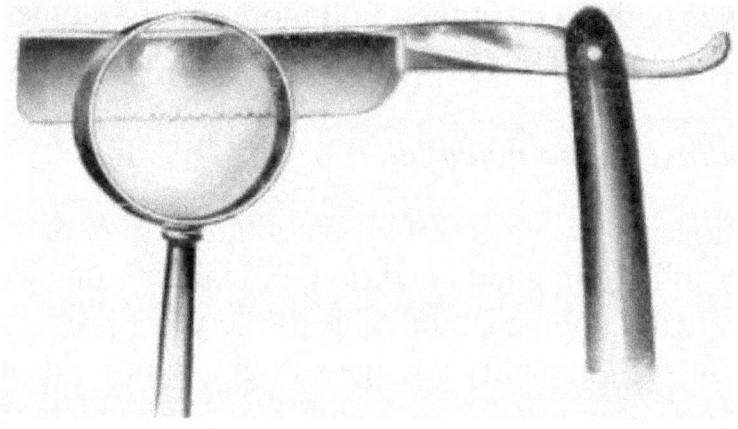

The edge of a straight razor as it would look under a microscope

These teeth run along the entire length of the blade and it is actually their microscopic size and the fact that these teeth occur regularly along the razor's edge, which makes a razor's edge exceedingly sharp. If these teeth become rounded or reduce in number then the razor becomes dull. To restore these teeth to their original condition it is, therefore, necessary to make the blade thinner, as simply stropping the blade cannot do this, it must be done by honing or sharpening the blade.

As many people these days only see a barber, preparing for a straight razor shave by stropping the blade many people don't realize that a straight razor like any out bladed tool will occasionally need to be sharpened, still others believe that once a razor's edge has been initially ground and set, stropping alone should be enough to keep a razor sharp. When one fully understands the individual roles the hone and strop play in keeping a straight razor's edge sharp one can plainly see that after many shaves stropping alone is not enough to keep a razor sharp.

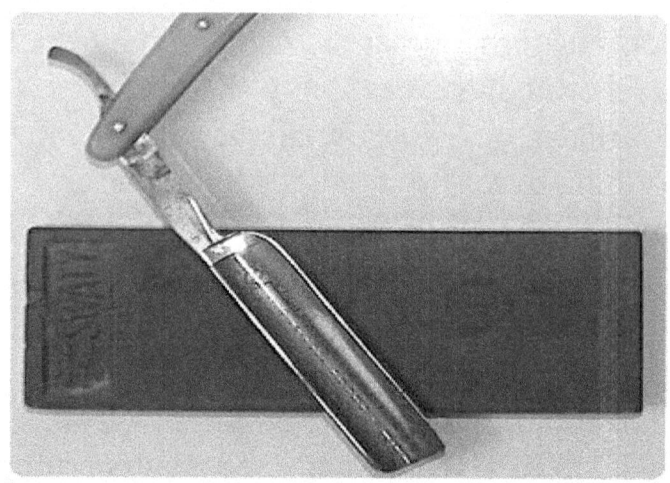

A Typical Razor Hone

The point of honing a razor is to make the edge as flat and thin as possible. This can only be done using a fine grit hone, which cuts and wears away the steel. A strop cannot do this. In fact the opposite is true, stropping a razor instead of giving it a thin, flat edge with a hone, will tend to further rounded the razor.

This is because the strop by its nature tends to sag whist stropping, and the more a strop is allowed to sag the quicker it will rounded the razor's edge and, therefore, the more you strop a dull blade the duller the blade will get. The flatter and thinner a razor's edge is the sharper it will be, and the only way to an archive a thin, flat blade is by honing it.

Before explaining how to hone a razor, I will explain the different types of hone available before you purchase one, this way you are armed with the knowledge you need to make an informed decision.

There are two main types of hone on the market, - one is a natural stone, which is cut from a natural rock, and the other is a man made or synthetic hone. Arguably, natural hones are best but finding the correct one can be confusing at best and expensive, and these days many a fine synthetic hone is produced in some ways; the synthetic hone are superior to natural stones as they are free of uneven spots and uniform in texture. These days the bulk of new hones used for sharpening straight razors come from Japan. I recommend a two-layered hone; the best I've found have a layer of 4000 grit on one side and an 8000 grit on the other side. I personally use and recommend Norton Japanese hone, but I'm sure there are many other fine hones out there.

Most beginners feel that honing is a difficult procedure and that expert barbers or cutlers should do it. Few feel they can sharpen their own razor. However, with the right knowledge and a suitable hone, honing a razor is as easy as stropping a razor and in the following chapter I will properly explain how this can be done.

How to Hone a Straight Razor

A hone is the only way to sharpen a razor, and it's imperative to use one if you intend to keep your razor in perfect condition.

Hones rarely are dry; instead they are normally covered with water, oil, or lather, the reasons being:

- To keep the blade cool, the process of honing creates heat, which could ruin the temper of the blade.
- To lubricate the surface of the hone making it easier to hone the blade and achieve a smother finish for the blade's edge.
- And to keep ground off partials of steel or swarf from blocking the pores of the stone, which would cause a glazed surface to be created on the stones surface.

With most hones you can either use lather, oil, or water, however, if you begin to hone with one never try to use another, if you start with oil continue to use oil in the future.

It takes more time to sharpen a razor using oil but the edge is smoother. If using water on the stone, it is best to submerge the stone in water for at least 15 minutes before you begin the process of honing.

Instructions for Honing

When honing, the hone should be placed on a flat solid surface.
The illustration below shows the exact pattern you should follow when honing a razor.

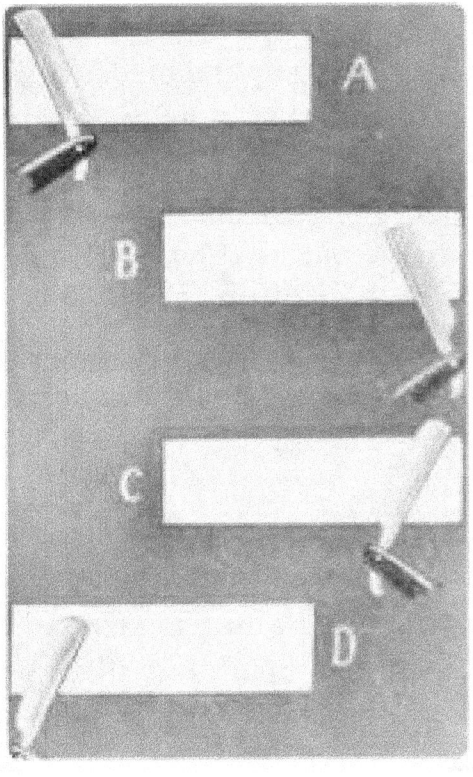

The Pattern You Should Follow When Honing Your Razor.

Figure A: So as to insure you have a firm hold of both the blade and the handle, with your thumb and fore finger holding the razor from the back of the heel. Now, drag the blade against the stone from heel to point, forward against the edge using a medium degree of pressure, until you get to *figure B*.

Figure B: Now, without lifting the blade from the hone, roll the blade over on its spine so the edge is now facing the opposite direction. Drag the blade forward this way till it rests in the position as indicted in *figure C*.

Figure C: Drag the blade from heel to point against the edge finishing the stroke as shown in *figure D*.

Figure D: Turn the blade on its back, slide from point to heel and by this stage you should be back to position shown in *figure A*.

Continue honing in this pattern until the blade is sufficiently sharp and free from any inequalities or nicks. You can determine this by drawing the edge, *very lightly*, across a moistened thumbnail. If it slightly sticks to the nail, this indicates that the razor is sufficiently honed and that the edge is now perfect.

If you have over-honed a "wire edge" would have developed and this must be remedied. To remedy this, *lightly* drag the edge across your moistened thumb as described previously. Now, drag the blade twice across the hone as before, in order to insure all parts of the blade are equal and that both sides of the blade are honed evenly.

Additional Instructions

The following are further considerations, which should be heeded whilst honing:

1. The blade should be honed perfectly flat to the stone, so that the spine and edge both are touching the stone. If the spine is raised while honing this will cause the blade to be honed blunt.

2. When dragging the blade across the hone diagonally against the edge, the heel should be about 1 ½ inches or 40mm forward of the point of the razor, and care take to insure this angle is maintained when the stroke is revised and throughout the procedure as this sets the microscopic teeth at their proper angle, which is slightly inclined toward the heel. The microscopic teeth on a straight razor are similar to that of a saw; however, the main difference between the two aside from size is that saw teeth incline away from the handle and toward the point, while the teeth of a straight razor point toward the heel. To

cut a saw one must push away from the handle toward the point, whereas a razor is usually drawn away from the point toward the heel.

Apply moderate and equal pressure on all parts of the edge. Very little pressure is needed if you are using a good hone.

The time it takes to properly hone a razor varies depending on the condition of the blade and the hardness of the steel it's made of. If the edge doesn't have any nicks and has become thick as a result of use or poor stropping then 8-10 strokes in each direction should be more then enough. If however, the edge has nicks, though some may be so small they can hardly be seen, this procedure will require more time and attention. If the nicks are large it is recommended that the razor be taken to a cutler to be properly ground.

If a straight razor is properly looked after and properly stropped, it should not frequently need honing, usually no more then once every six months. If the razor requires honing you will know as stropping will not sharpen it.

The Strop

The reason we hone a razor is to thin and true up the blade. However, once this has been done, the process of sharpening the razor is still not complete, because the edge whilst being honed was left rough and unfit for shaving. The point of stropping in this process is not to thin the edge, but to smooth the edge, removing the rough surface of the microscopic teeth that were developed during the honing process, and setting them in perfect alignment. This is what makes a straight razor extremely sharp.

For this, you should use a top quality strop. If your strop is of poor quality or is rough or worn, then it makes little difference how good the razor itself is it will be impossible to keep the razor in shave worthy condition. It is quite common for a razor to be blamed for a poor shave when the fault lies with the strop and how it has been used. It is recommended to use chromium oxide paste with your strop, however this should be used sparingly as over use may actually wear down the microscopic teeth and gradually ruin the temper of the steel.

There are currently many types of strops on the market, some are of excellent quality and some are absolute junk. The most common strop on the market is the swing strop, which features leather on one side and rubber on the other. Some cheaper strops use lower quality canvas or leather, which may ruin your razor and should be avoided.

A good leather strop should be enough but if you wish to use a combination strop the rubber or canvas side should be of the best quality.

The strop should be at least two inches wide and twenty inches long. Make sure the surface is smooth and soft and not glazed, you can tell weather the surface is by rubbing your hand over it.

Never fold a strop when you are storing it, as it is likely that you will roughen or crack the surface, and this may adversely affect the edge of your razor when you next strop it.

Caring For Your Strop

After a strop has been used a lot it may sometimes be found to have lost its "cling", which means the blade will feel slippery while stropping, therefore, it will fail to provide a sharp, smooth cutting edge to the blade. The reason for this is that the strop has dried out and become porous. To remedy this hang the strop on a hook, and with the left-hand light stretch. Apply a good thick lather to the surface of the strop and use your hand to massage it in. What the strop needs is to have it pores filled with lather so keep applying and massaging in coats of lather until the pores of the strop can hold no more lather. Then allow the strop to dry. This treatment will rejuvenate the strop, and the next time you use it you will be pleasantly surprised to note its improved effect on the razor as the "cling" will have been restored.

How To Strop Your Razor

Make sure you hook your razor to something firmly mounted and that it is positioned about four to five feet off the ground. With your left hand firmly hold the handle as demonstrated in the illustration below.

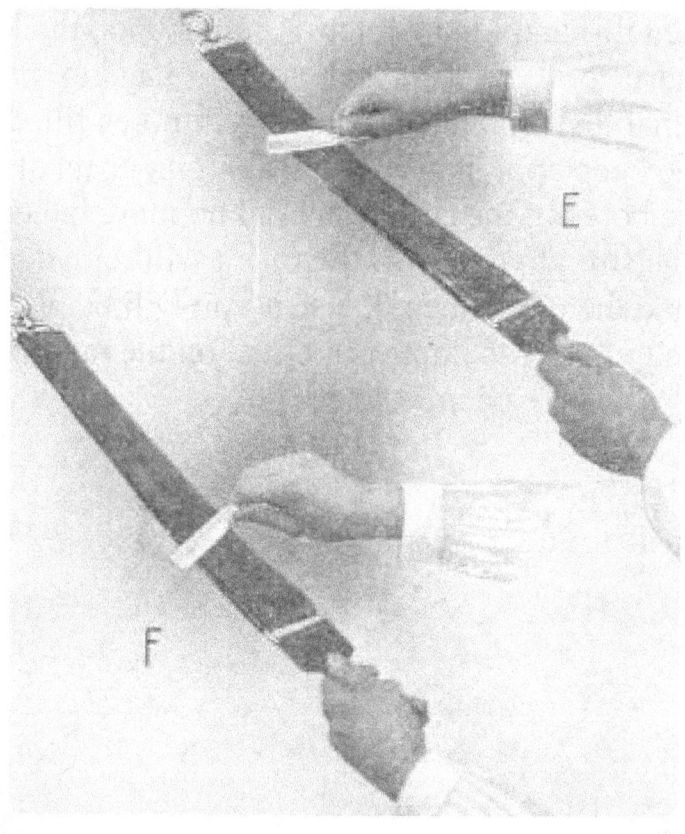

How to Strop Your razor.

Pull the strop tight, never allow a strop to hang as this will cause the edge of the razor to become rounded and thus will need to be re-honed.

Open the razor, so the handle is in line with the blade. Hold the razor firmly with your right hand, with the first two fingers and thumb holding the razor just behind the heel, as this will give you complete control of both the handle and the blade. With the razor held like this it is easier to roll the razor back and forth from one side to another.

Lay the blade flat on the furthest end of the strop, as demonstrated in *figure E,* with the razors edge away from you. Draw the blade back toward you, always keeping the heel of the razor forward of the point. When the razor has reached the back end of the strop, roll the razor until the un-stropped side of the blade makes contact with the strop as demonstrated in *figure F.* Now with the heel behind the point, push the razor away from you until it reaches the furthest end of the strop. Again roll the razor, and continue stropping until the razor is properly sharpened.

Always hold the razor at the same angle and perfectly flat on the strop. Always strop in the opposite direction used in honing. NEVER strop in the same direction as the razor will snag the strop and damage the strop and the razor's edge. In honing, the heel is always forward of the point and in stropping it is always back. As with honing, during stropping the back of the razor must always be in contact with the strop.

By doing this and always rolling the blade on its spine you will avoid damaging the strop or the razor. If you have just started learning take your time and strop slowly until you become proficient.

If the razor's edge is in good condition and not in need of honing fifteen to twenty passes in each direction should be sufficient. However, if the razor does require honing, no amount of stropping will sharpen it.

Because a razor's edge does oxidize in short order and picks up microscopic rust partials it is advisable to also strop your razor before every shave.

The Shaving Mug

These days there is a wide variety of shaving mugs available made from a wide variety of materials and of various shapes and sizes that choosing the right mug can be difficult and confusing.

When selecting a shaving mug, make sure the mug is big enough to accommodate the shaving soap and with a mouth big enough to allow you to create a good lather with your brush.

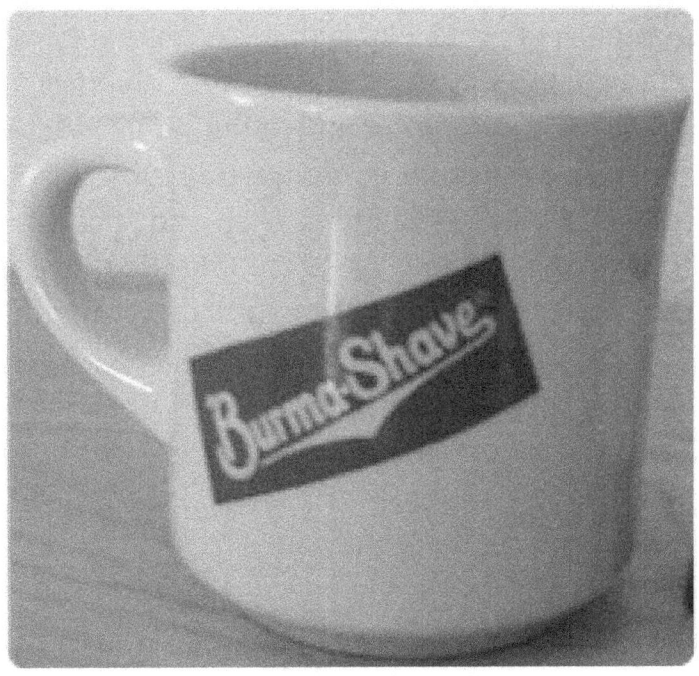

Typical Shaving Mug

Where possible the soap should completely fill the base of you mug with no room to move around or else water will get in between the base of the mug and the bottom of the soap. If you find the cake of soap doesn't completely fill the base of the mug the easiest way to solve this problem is to take the soap out of the mug and warm it until it become slightly soft, place the cake back in the mug and then using your hand press the sides of the cake, thereby flattening it out until it fills the empty gaps between the edge of the soap and the side of the mug. If at any time the soap dislodges from the bottom of the mug it should be pressed back in place as soon as possible.

You should always make sure that the mug is kept completely clean. Rinsing it out completely after shaving, to make sure you remove any unused lather. Make sure the mug is not contaminated with dust. Some men use sticks of shaving soap and shaving foam from a can or tube. While these are OK, I believe it is better to make the lather in a cup and apply it with a brush.

The Soap

Second to the razor the right shaving soap is most important item in your shaving kit. Properly applied quality soap is the secret to an easy, comfortable shave especially with a straight razor. No matter, how good your razor is, unless the face is properly lathered with a good quality soap, you shave will be anything but comfortable.

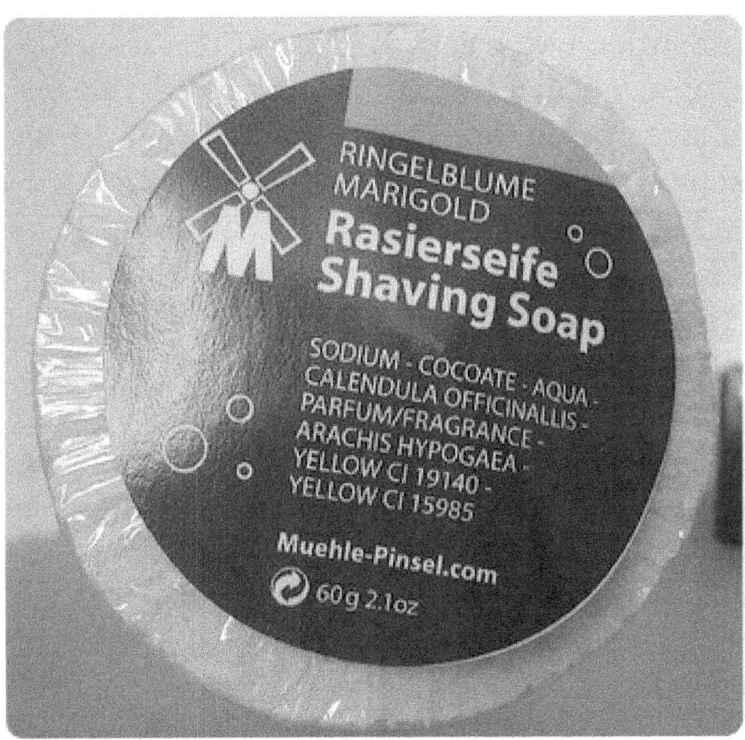

A Cake of Traditional Shaving Soap

Only, use a recognized brand of soap, specifically designed for shaving, under no circumstances should you use regular bath soap for shaving. The lather is not suitable for shaving and will more then likely dry and irritate the skin and leave your face sore and rough.

Most people have the wrong idea regarding the use of soap. The most prevalent idea regarding the use of soap is that the purpose of using soap is to soften the facial hair, in order to make it easier to cut. This is a fallacy. The exact opposite is true, the soap is designed to make the hair stiffer, brittle and protrude further from the skin so that it will become firmer and more resistant against the surface of the razor. It is common knowledge that hair is tube comprised of a hard fibrous matter, growing from a bulb under the surface of the skin also known as a follicle, which also secretes bodily oil. This oil works it's way up through the hair, and by permeating all parts of the hair makes the hair softer. Now due to this oily condition makes it very difficult to cut the hair with a razor, and it become even more difficult for the hair is made softer due to the application of hot water. Many men do this and understandably find shaving more difficult. When hot water is applied the hairs become limp and soft, and the razor will either skip over them, bend them back, slice them lengthwise or partly cut into while also pulling them at the roots, thereby making shaving a more uncomfortable experience and promoting skin irritation. Shaving soap has the opposite effect.

Shaving soap usually contains either an alkali, soda or potash which when lathered up and applied to the facial hair neutralizes the oil or removes it therefore, causing the hair to become stiff and brittle and in this condition they may be easily cut by the razor. Of course, for the sake of hygiene, you should wash your face to remove any dirt or dead skin cells from the facial hair; but prior to lathering you should dry your face with a towel.

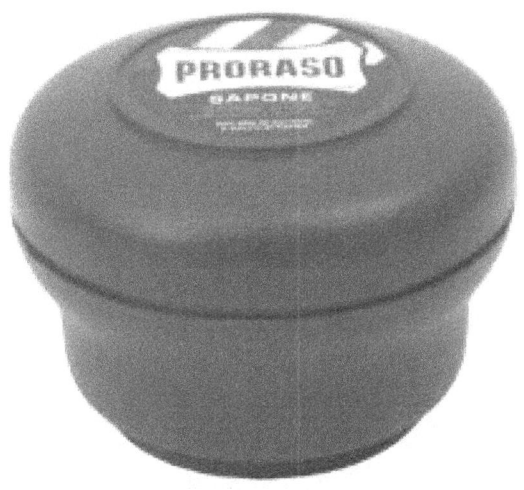

For people who cannot be bothered using a traditional shave with a traditional mug and soap but would still like a traditional shave, many shaving soap companies offer their soap cake complete with container as shown in the above illustration which acts as a mug and the lid acts to prevent duct and dirt contaminating the soap the last one I used lasted me over a year.

The Shaving Brush

Most shaving brushes, which are commonly available, can have a variety of bristles. The most common types of bristle available for shaving brushes are badger hair, boar hair, are man made bristles or can be a combination of all three. The best shaving brushes are generally made of 100% badger hair.

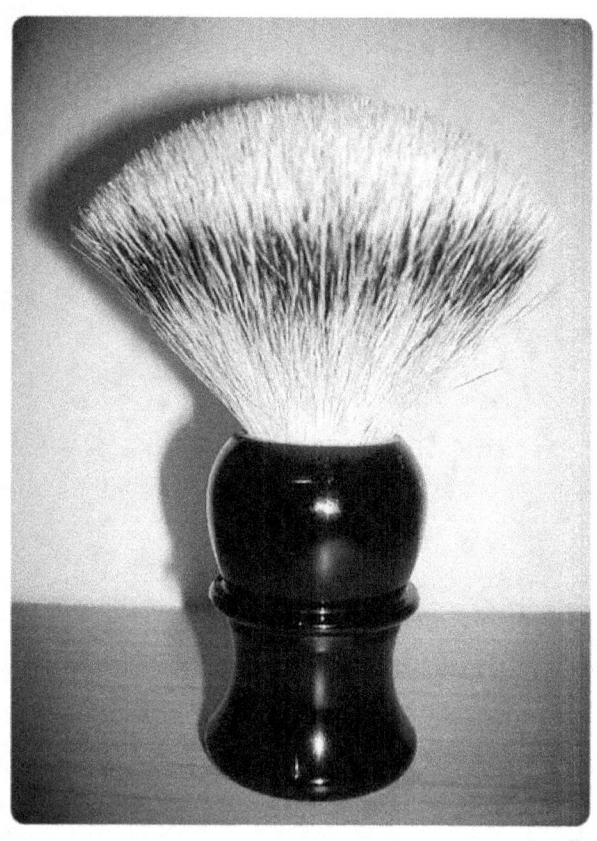

With shaving brushes it is best to always buy the best you can find, on the outside there is little apparent difference between a poor quality brush and a good quality brush.

The bristles of a cheap brush are usually set into the base with cement, glue or resin, which usually cracks in short order in which case the bristles start falling out.

A good quality brush is usually set in hard rubber which with proper care will last for years, Also, a poor quality brush won't lather up as well as a good brush and as good brush usually doesn't cost much more then a poor quality brush in the long run a good quality brush works out to be cheaper.

Caring for Your Shaving Brush.

After using a shaving brush NEVER leave lather to dry on it, after shaving thoroughly rinse it with hot water and dry the brush with a towel. It is also good practice to hang a shaving brush upside down to air dry before storing it.

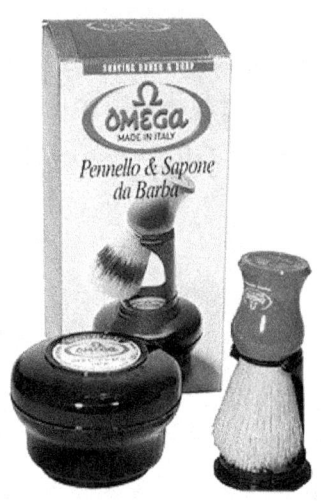

A shave set such as the one above may be an ideal starting point for a beginner, as it does away with the need to purchase a mug, soap and brush separately as everything is included in the set, also a shave set like this comes with a rack which allows you to hang the brush upside down to dry, thereby , greatly extending the life of the brush.

How to Create a Good Lather

To create a good lather, insure the soap is placed in the mug according to the previous instructions. Fill the mug with warm water, allow it to sit for a few seconds, now tip the all water out. There should be enough water residues inside the mug to make a lather, which will adhere to the mug, brush and soap. Now, using the brush, stir thoroughly using a churning action, until you get a good thick lather. The more you rub the brush over the soap the thicker the lather should become. A lot depends on having a lather of a correct consistency. If the lather is runny and thin, you will a poor shave. The creamer the lather is the better it will stiffen the hairs. In fact, the lather should have a consistency similar to that of whipped cream. Some lower quality soaps will very quickly produce lather, however it will be found to be thin and watery.

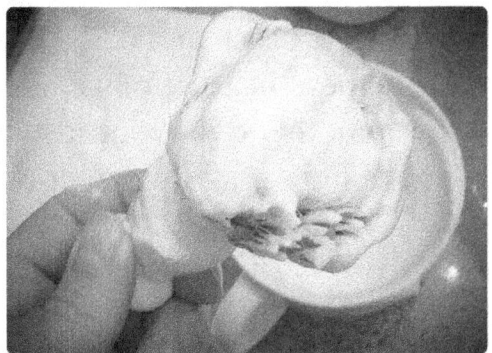

Illustration above shows what a good lather should look like.

So that by the time you have shaved one side of your face the lather has all but run off the other side. A good soap will create a thick lather that will last the entire shaving process.

How to Apply the Lather

Apply the lather with the brush and cover every part of your face, which you intend to shave. Use the brush's bristles to thoroughly work the lather into your beard until the lather has had enough time to stiffen the facial hair. This step is imperative to a good shave as it is impossible to have easily shaved unless the face is well lather and the lather has been worked into the beard. Now, go over your face once more with your shaving brush and spread the lather over your face evenly, and begin shaving immediately before the lather has had a chance to dry. If the lather dries before you have finished shaving, slightly wet the brush and add some fresh lather. If you follow these instructions closely, a sharp razor will slide so smoothly over your face that shaving will be a pleasurable and satisfying experience.

How to Handle Your Straight Razor

If you are just learning how to shave with a straight razor it is imperative the to learn the right way from the beginning. You can just as easily learn the wrong way to do anything in life as you can learn the right way. I know putting that cold, sharp straight razor close to your face for the first time can be daunting. Maybe before this you have tried and failed, but as Henry Ford once said "failure is just the opportunity to start again, this time more intelligently". And, I'm certain if you follow the instructions contained in this book closely, with practice and dedication you will have no difficulty in learning how to comfortably and safely shave yourself with a straight razor.

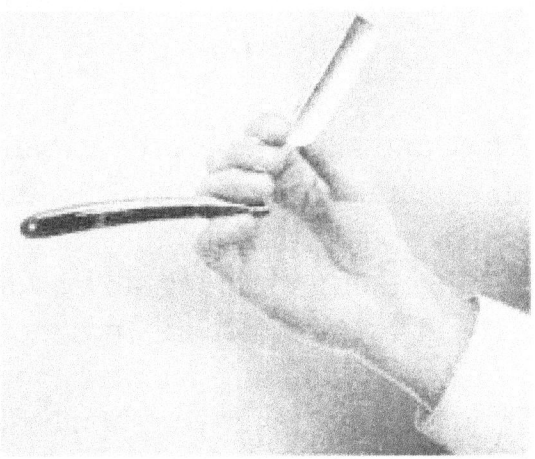

The Correct Way to Hold a Straight Razor.

The illustration on the previous page shows the correct position in which to hold a straight razor. Before holding the razor in preparation for shaving make sure your hands are dry and are NOT slippery. You should observe the scales are kicked back over the heel of the razor. The first the fingers rest on the back of the blade, with the thumb near the middle, on the other side of the blade and the little one over the hook at on the end. You will be in complete control of your razor in this position as the scales act as a counter balance and there will be little chance of cutting yourself. This basic position should change little throughout the process of shaving, although you may find it necessary to change this position slightly whilst shaving certain parts of your face such as under your jaw or neck. But whatever position you shave it is imperative you maintain control of the razor at all times.

The Stroke

Everybody's face and hair type is different and, therefore the manner in which you shave with your straight razor is as individual as you. Some men find short quick strokes best while other prefer long slow strokes. Each man must shave in a way, which he finds most comfortable. However certain principles apply to everyone. If you are a beginner you should start of slowly and gradually increase you speed as you become more proficient and comfortable. As you become more familiar with shaving with a straight razor you will develop more speed without even realizing.

Hold the razor relatively flat to your face at an approximate 30 degree angle to the skin.

Shave in the direction grain not against it as shown in the illustration below:

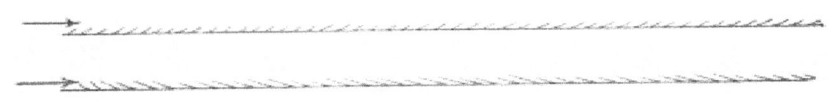

Shaving against the grain pulls against the hair, irritates the skin can cause ingrown hairs and if the facial hair is long and stiff can cause the blade to catch the hairs and be deflected upward or inward and cause you to cut your face and NEVER under any circumstances try to shave against the grain when shaving your upper lip.

How to Position Your Mirror

When shaving in front of a mirror the mirror should be positioned in a well-lit area so you can get a good reflection of all sides of your face. The mirror should be at a height, which makes it comfortable and ergonomic for you to shave.

It is also good practice to either remove your shirt or place a towel around you neck to avoid soiling your cloths.

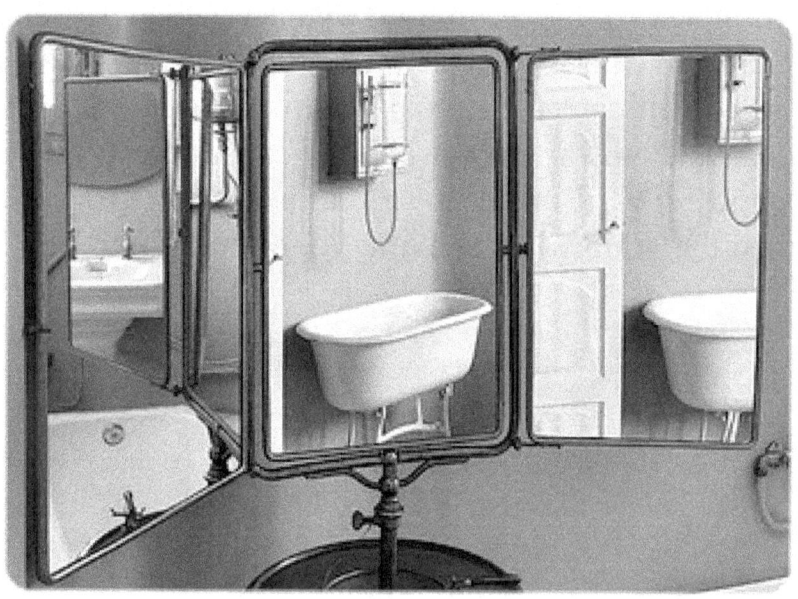

How To Correctly Shave with A Straight Razor

To simplify the process of shaving with a straight razor as much as possible this section has been broken down into 6 detailed steps.

Step 1.

How to Right Side of Your Face Above the Jaw Line.

- Reach your left hand over your head and with your fingers positioned just above your right side-burn pull skin upward, thus creating a smooth surface on which to shave.

- Shave in a downward direction until about half of you right cheek has been shaved.

- Slide your left hand further over until your fingers are positioned in the middle of your cheek and again pull your skin upward.

- Now continue to shave in a downward direction until your entire face is shaved to the middle of your chin and well under your jaw line.

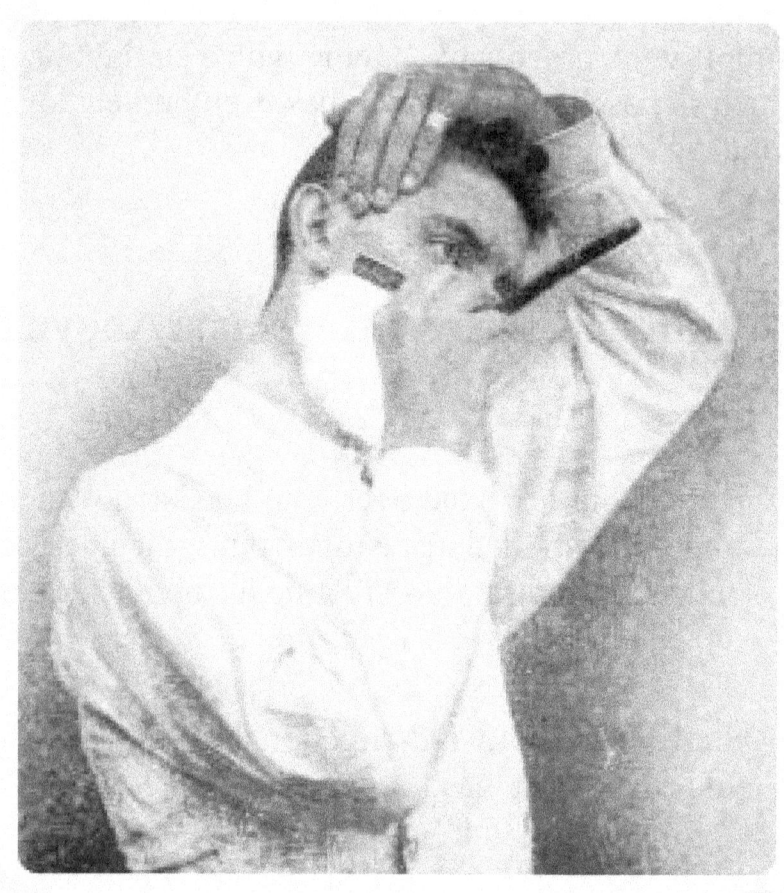

Illustration above shows the correct position for shaving above the right side of your jaw line.

Step 2.

How to Shave the Right Side of Your Face Below the Jaw Line

- Tilt your head toward the left side and keep your chin slightly elevated.

- With the fingers of your left hand, pull your skin tight under the jaw

- If your beard grows downward shave in a downward direction; if it doesn't, revise the stroke.

- Unless, it cannot be avoided you should never shave against the grain on your first pass.

Keep your skin pulled and tightly as possible as this will create a smoother shaving surface and reduce the risk of cutting yourself.

The illustration on the next page shows the correct position for this step.

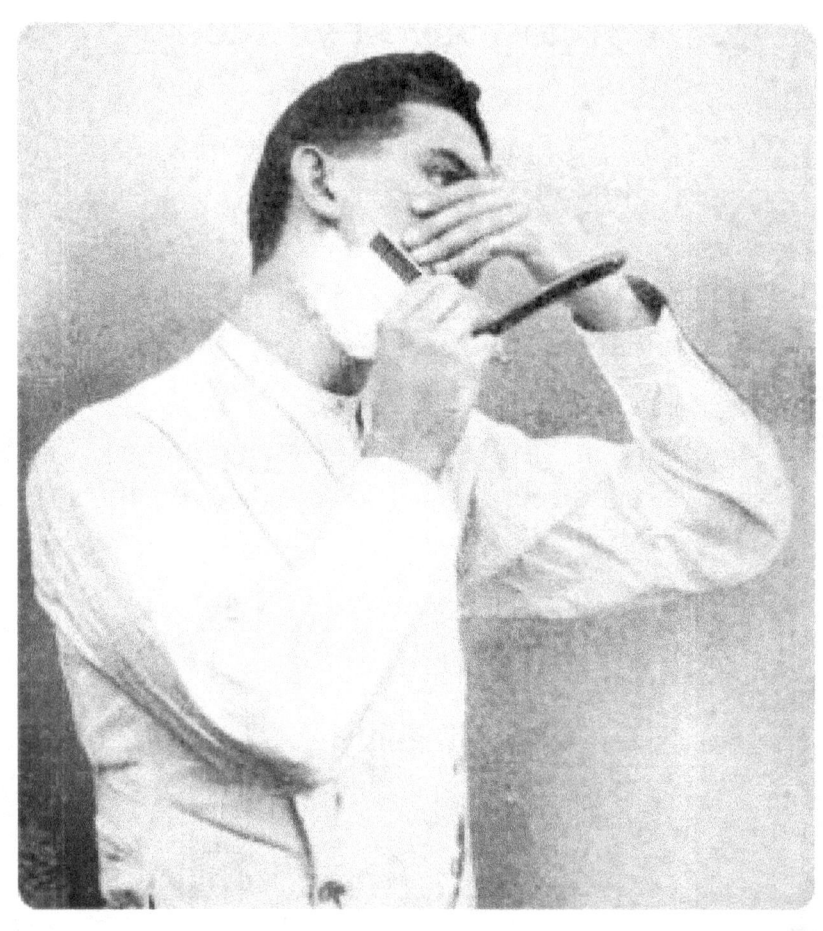

Illustration above shows the correct position for shaving below the right side of your jaw line.

Step 3.

How to Left Side of Your Face Above the Jaw Line

- Place the fingers of your left hand in front of and just above your left ear and press in an upward direction to pull the skin of your upper left cheek smooth

- With the razor's toe pointing upward and with the razor in your right hand, reach across your face and shave in a downward motion.

- When shaving the lower part of you cheek and chin, follow downward with your left hand, keeping the skin tightly pulled back. To shave your upper lip, draw your lip down to tighten the skin and move you nose out of way. Because of the muscle in your lip, you shouldn't have to use your left hand for this.

The illustration on the next page shows the correct position for this step.

47

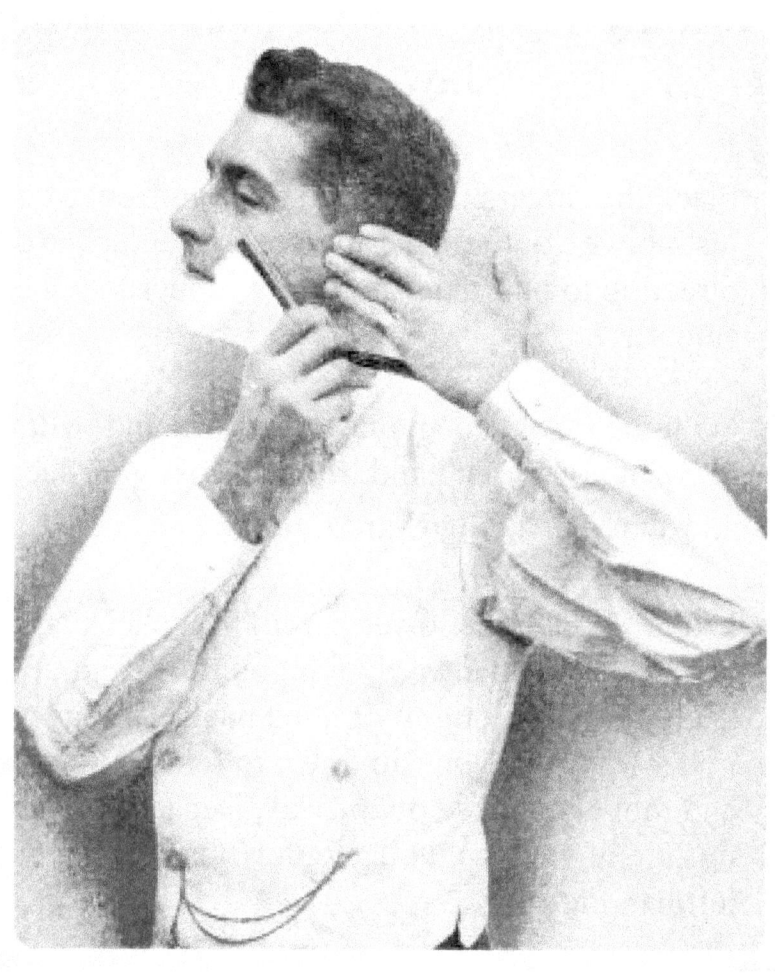

Illustration above shows the correct position for shaving the left side of your face above jaw line.

Step 4.

How to Shave the Left Side of Your Face Below the Jaw Line

For lots of men this is the hardest part to shave because the skin in this area is very sensitive and unless treated delicately tends to become sore and irritated. To easily shave this area:

- Tilt your head to the right and raise your chin.

- Using your left hand pull the skin back a tightly as possible from the base of your neck.

- Shave in a downward direction, unless your facial hair grows in the opposite direction in this case you should reverse the stroke.

The illustration on the next page shows the correct position for this step.

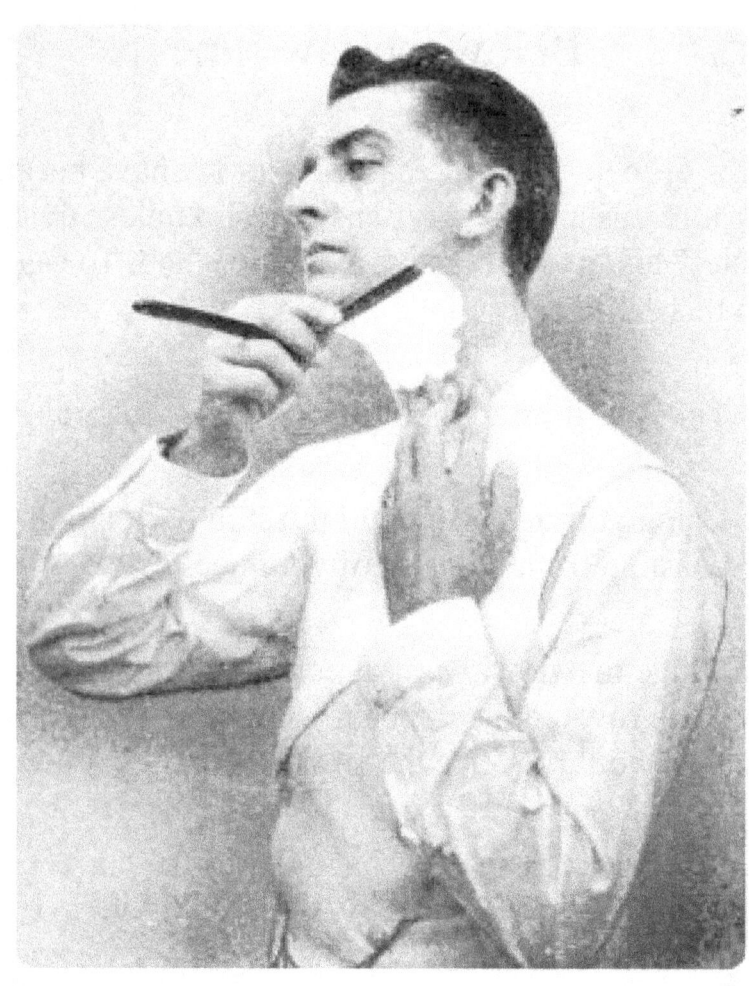

Illustration above shows the correct position the left side of your face below the jaw line.

Step 5.

How to Shave Under Your Chin

- Tilt you head backward to raise your chin.

- Holding the razor with your right hand and using the fingers of your left hand pull the skin downward from the base of your neck.

The illustration below shows the correct position for this step.

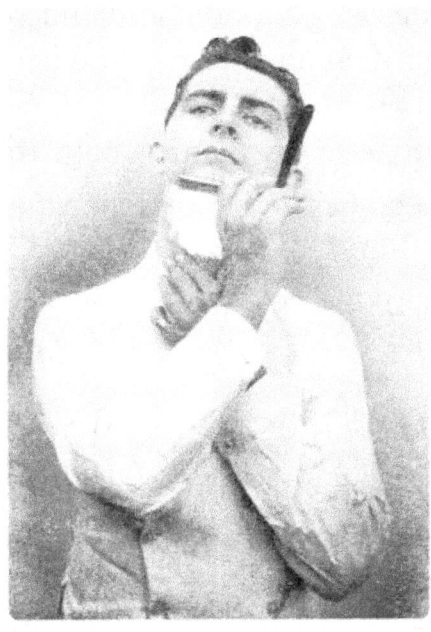

Step 6.

The Second Pass

If you truly want a clean shave, you will need to shave your face a second time. Strop your razor a few more times before beginning and lather your face again. Instead of shaving with the grain, many men, when doing a second pass, like to reverse the stroke and shave against the grain. This can give a much closer shave then shaving with the grain, however if your facial hair is thick and heavy or you have sensitive skin this may cause skin irritation and may cause in grown hairs. Again NEVER use this method when shaving the upper lip. If you are a beginner, I would recommend you shave with the grain instead if against it until you become more proficient.
However, it is up to every man to make this decision on his own circumstances and experience.

The illustration on the next page shows how to shave against the grain.

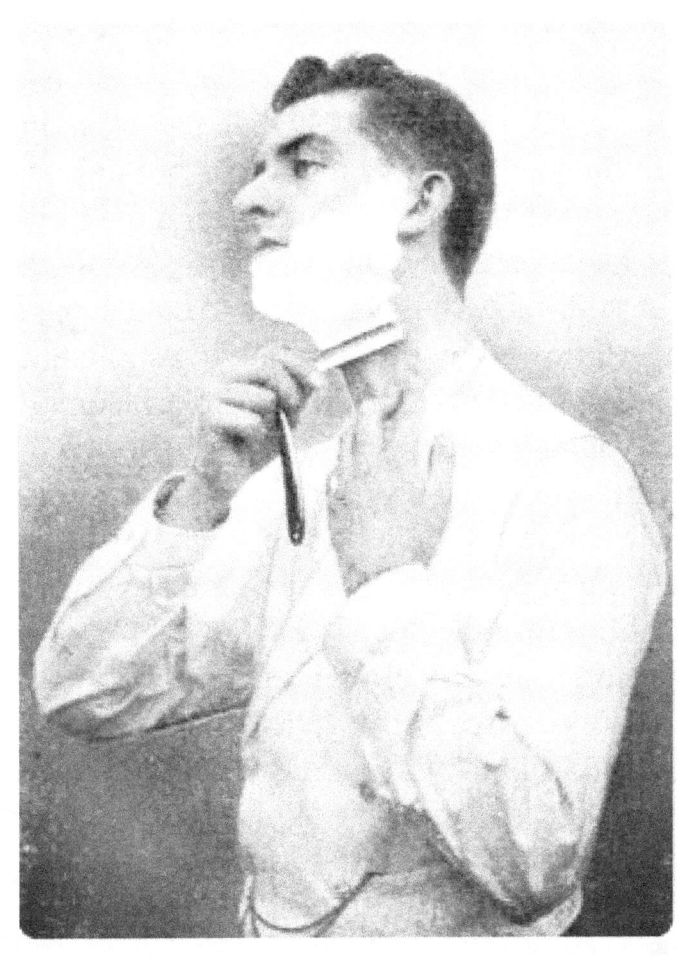

Illustration above shows how to shave against the grain.

Treating Your Face After Shaving

Many men seem think that after they have shaving that, they have finished the job and there is nothing further to. This is wrong, as they do not understand the importance of proper facial care. The quickest and easiest way to look after your face after a shave is to splash on some aftershave followed by evenly applying some talcum or baby powder. Most men would just splash some aftershave on and be done.

To keep the skin in healthy condition a little extra, elaborate treatment should be confided. I recommend, after washing your face after shaving that you apply a steaming hot towel (as hot as you can stand) to your face. The hot, moist towel will open your pores and draw the blood to your face. Now apply your favorite aftershave and finally, thoroughly massage your face. This is very beneficial for the skin. Many men suffer from slugging blood flow to the scalp and face due the slow heart action and as result the many small vanes under the surface of the skin become blocked. Massaging the skin encourages the blood to flow close to the surface of the skin, filling the many minuscule vanes just below the surface of the skin. You face will thank you for this, as your face will really feel invigorated and fresh.

How to Treat a Cut

These are six main reasons as to why a man may occasionally cut himself while shaving, which are:

1. Trying to shave with a blunt razor and applying more force then would be otherwise needed if the razor was sufficiently sharp.

2. Trying to shave with a razor with to thin a blade, which bend and springs on the face.

3. Trying to shave with a razor, which has a sharp point.

4. Shaving in a hurry, (relax and enjoy the experience).

5. Shaving against the grain.

6. Not holding the razor properly or using the razor in a careless manner

You will rarely cut or nick yourself if you avoid the above mistakes and exercise common sense. But if you do cut your self you should know how to treat the cut. If it is only small nick, applying pressure to the cut or covering the cut with a towel and holding in place for a little while can sometimes stop the bleeding.

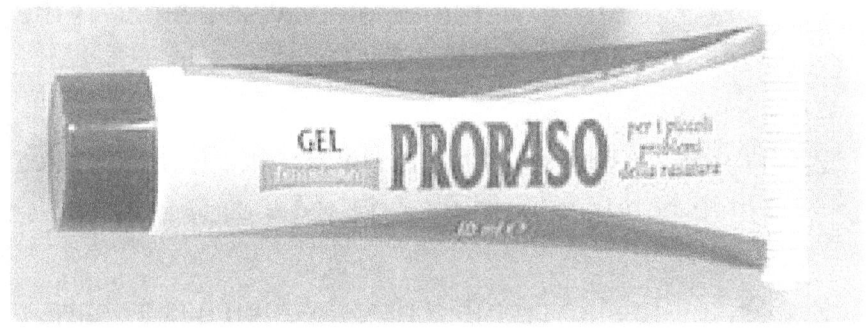

Barber's Styptic Gel

If this doesn't stop the bleeding, use an astringent or some type of antiseptic. Styptic pencils or styptic gel are specifically designed for this purpose. You don't happen to have any styptic gel in your bathroom cabinet? Try using some Listerine if it was good enough for cleaning wounds on the battlefield in World War 1 it's good enough to clean your little shaving nick. If you do cut your self don't get discouraged it happens to even the most experienced straight razor user from time to time.

The Causes of Skin Irritation and How It Can Be Prevented

After shaving many men suffer from skin irritation and razor burn. This section is dedicated for these men in the hope that the suggestions out lined here will help or, if not entirely prevent this discomfort.

The main cause of skin irritation is a blunt razor. When a razor is sharp it will easily cut the hairs with minimal passes required therefore, producing little or no irritation. However, if the razor is blunt, rather then slicing through the hairs easily, it will slice some lengthwise, pass over others and generally strain and pull at the roots of the hair. This means having to pass over the same area over and over again, to get a reasonable shave, which can result in irritated skin, which can last until you next shave and repeat the uncomfortable procedure again. Thus, some men suffer from continual irritation. The easiest way to remedy this problem is to ensure your razor is always sharp and in prime condition.

Shaving too close may be another cause, and men who believe this could be the cause should consider shaving with on pass instead of two.

Not every man's skin is the same so therefore, it stands to reason that not all aftershaves will suit all skin types. Many alcohol-based aftershaves can irritate sensitive skin. These days there are many alcohol free aftershaves on the market. So it might be worthwhile to try another brand of aftershave.

Sometimes the problem could be the quality of the shaving soap you are using. I personally had this problem when I used to use aerosol-shaving foams and gels, these days I only use the best traditional styles soap I can find, usually I use Proraso.

After shaving make sure you wash you face thoroughly and leave no trace of lather on you face it's a good idea after shaving to wipe you face with a steaming hot towel as discussed previously in this book.

Some men experience irritation more then others. Men with heavy stiff facial hair and tender skin and more susceptible then others, however, with proper care skin most irritations can be avoided.

Of course if the problems persist it is recommended to speak with a dermatologist.

The End.